The

MW01518871

Gym Marketing Secrets:

A No-Fluff And Comprehensive Manual
For Gym Owners Who Want
More Leads And More Clients

by Mark Fisher

businessforunicorns.com
@businessforunicorns

The Little Book of Gym Marketing Secrets:
A No-Fluff And Comprehensive Manual For Gym Owners
Who Want More Leads And More Clients

Copyright © **2024 Business for Unicorns**

ISBN: 979-8-218-44089-3

All Rights Reserved.

No part of this book may be reproduced or transmitted in any form by any means, electronic or mechanical, including photocopying, recording, or by any information storage and retrieval system, without prior written permission from the author.

All translations of this work must be approved in writing by the author. Please contact Business for Unicorns for permission to translate and distribution agreements.

Printed in the United States of America.

For more, go to:
GymMarketingSecretsBook.com
BusinessForUnicorns.com

First Edition

Hey there fellow Gym Owner!

Let's come right out with it: marketing a gym can be hard.

It's frustrating when…

- Your lead flow is more like a lead trickle
- You're doing lots of "marketing stuff," but not getting traction
- Your sales opportunities are wildly inconsistent from week to week

What we want is:

- A steady stream of interested — and qualified — prospects
- The peace of mind that comes from knowing we're using our time well
- A growing base of happy clients and revenue that increases month over month

In this book, you'll learn the very best tools and strategies for achieving these goals.

We will cover:

- Core Marketing Tools
- Lead Generation Systems
- Lead Nurture Systems
- Lead Conversion Systems
- Marketing Planners

This short book is going to be dense and devoid of any fluff. Buckle up! ;-)

A BIT ABOUT YOUR AUTHOR

Before we dig in, I think it's prudent to ask a bit more about my credentials.

Or… *"Who the F is this guy?"* ;-)

My name is Mark Fisher. I'm a co-founder of **Business for Unicorns**. We help gym owners create more income, more impact, and more freedom.

And I don't just talk about the gym business. I also own and operate gyms myself, including NYC's eccentric Mark Fisher Fitness.

MFF has been on the Inc 500 as one of the fastest growing companies in America. We've also been named one of Men's Health's Top Gyms in America. We've been featured in *The New York Times, Forbes, the Wall St Journal, DETAILS, Fox News, CBS News,* and many other media outlets. We've done well over $35 million in revenue since opening in 2012.

Thanks to MFF and BFU, I've had the chance to speak and travel all over the world. I've given talks and keynotes for Perform Better, IDEA, FILEX, the Fitness Business Summit, Anytime Fitness Australia, Mike Boyle Strength & Conditioning, SCW Mania, Camp Gladiator, and many, many more.

I've coached and consulted with household name brands both in and out of fitness. I've worked with massive fitness franchises (including as a franchisee myself), scores of mom-and-pop independent gyms, and everything in between. I'm also a gym business book author, YouTube creator, and podcaster. And most of all? I'm a lifelong learner who's an operator at heart. And I LOVE gyms. :-)

If you want to know more about me or Business for Unicorns, here are some places to check us out:

- BusinessForUnicorns.com
- MarkFisherYouTube.com
- BFUPodcast.com
- BusinessForUnicorns.com/Book

The last URL will take you to another book I wrote. It's a bunch of lessons and stories from my 10-plus years running MFF.

And if you want a FREE digital copy?

Message us on Instagram at **@businessforunicorns** and we'll get you one!

SPECIAL OFFER

I've written this little book to show you exactly how to get more leads and more clients. But I know you're not really looking to just read a book. You want results.

And I know some percentage of readers will want more support to *go faster*. #marketing

I'd love to invite you to a *free 10-minute brainstorming session* with me or someone on my team.

In this fast-paced call, we'll get clear on:

- The specific results you want in the next 90 days and beyond
- The #1 roadblock restricting your growth and holding you back
- A clear 3-Step Plan to get you results in your gym ASAP

*Go to **BusinessForUnicorns.com/Brainstorm***

OR use the QR code below to book your call today.

CORE MARKETING TOOLS

These tools are the foundation of your marketing and sales efforts. You'll clarify your dream client. You'll build a compelling website and offer designed just for them. And you'll finalize the numbers to track and assess your results.

☐ Metrics Dashboard

Most gym owners don't find numbers sexy. But in the game of business, this is how we keep score.

The good news is we don't want an overly complicated dashboard. More mature gyms benefit from some weekly targets. But in the beginning, it may be best to track monthly.

Once per week, you'll update your most important numbers with your month-to-date results. This will clarify how you're doing compared to your goals. We don't want to wait until the 27th of a given month to find you've only had 3 leads all month long.

Suggested Metrics:

- Leads
- Trials (also called Front End Offers or Low Barrier Offers)
- Sales Appointments
- New Members
- Active Clients (on the 1st of the month)
- Terminations
- Churn %

☐ Client Avatar Worksheet

This is a simple document that paints a crystal clear picture of your dream client. Your worksheet will clarify two kinds of information:

- *Demographics* (age, fitness background, job, income, hobbies, etc.)
- *Psychographics* (frustrations, fears, wants, aspirations, etc.)

The more specific you can be, the better. All your marketing should be designed to attract your dream client.

You can use the *demographic information* to identify:

- Where your dream client hangs out
- What organizations they belong to
- What media they consume
- What events they attend
- What other businesses they patronize
- And more

This will help you decide where to market so you can find your dream clients.

The *psychographic information* will inform all marketing copy. It will help you enter the conversation already going on in their head, in the words they actually use.

Finally, tailor your brand's visual design and feel to be highly attractive to your avatar.

☐ **Gym Website**

Your website should have a headline and call to action that makes it immediately clear:

> 1) WHO you help
> 2) HOW you help them
> 3) Exactly what they should DO next

A good headline framework is:

We help [This kind of person] [Achieve this kind of result].

Your "call to action" (what you want them to DO) should drive to a button "above the fold" (meaning you don't have to scroll down). The button should visually "pop" and use text that makes it very clear what to do next. You can't be too obvious here.

Examples include:

- *Claim Your Free Workout*
- *Talk to a Trainer*
- *Book a Free Intro*
- *Claim Your X-Day Challenge*

Use compelling pictures of real people working hard and enjoying the process. These pics should highlight people your avatar finds both relatable AND aspirational.

In addition to your homepage, consider having:

- A Testimonials page for case studies and testimonials
- An About Us page that provides more details about your services and/or background

Just remember, the website has one goal: *get visitors to take action.* The primary CTA is taking the first step to book your front end offer. You can also have a "secondary" CTA lower down on the homepage that offers a valuable resource in exchange for their email address.

BONUS: Download speed matters for Google search rankings AND conversions. Use a site like GTMetrix.com to test your site.

Finally, although it's not your website, don't forget to optimize your **Google Business Profile**. This will make it easier for prospects to find you when searching for gyms in the area. At the very least, keep your hours up to date and periodically post new pictures. Strive to add a new post at least a couple of times per month. And ALWAYS leave a response to all Google Reviews.

☐ Front End Offer

Your gym will need a high-value offer that prospects actually want. A good first offer has minimal risk and makes it easy to get started with you.

The best offer will vary based on your services. Most gyms do best offering a "low barrier offer" that makes it very easy to get started. in general, a good low barrier offer looks like this:

- 14-30 days
- 3+ sessions per week
- Under $100
- 100% No-Hassle Money Back Guarantee
- A name (e.g. *Name of Gym Kickstart, Name of Gym Challenge, etc.*)
- A Strategy Session where you will sell them the best membership for their goals

Most gyms do best driving prospects to a 10-minute Discovery Call to sell their front end offer. In this case, you can also charge more (up to $600+ if you position it as a high-value transformation offer).

Alternatively, if it's less than $100, you can test selling it directly on your website. If you go this route, be sure to make it very easy to buy. Use Stripe if possible. You may need to manually link their credits to your booking and billing platform. But it's worth it for them to be able to buy via ApplePay double-click on their phone.

After purchase, the next step is a 10-minute Discovery Call OR a 30-45 minute Strategy Session. This is where you'll handle any logistics and start the sales process. (Check out the **Lead Conversion Systems** section later in the book for more on these.)

Some related tools you'll need:

- [ ] Calendar software to book a Discovery Call
- [ ] Landing page to host Discovery Call calendar

    - This page needs a benefit rich headline, clear CTA, and calendar above-the-fold

- [ ] Low Barrier Offer Product built in your booking billing software
- [ ] Landing page for prospects to buy (OPTIONAL and only if clients buy on their own)

PRO TIP: "Gate" the booking calendar. Get their first name, phone number, and email *first*. This way you can automate a text and email follow-up with prospects who don't finish the booking process. You can also be alerted to call them as soon as possible.

LEAD GENERATION SYSTEMS

You've now clarified exactly who you work with and what leads should do next. Now we'll need systems to generate leads and grow your audience of prospects.

Marketing and sales progress through three steps:

- **KNOW** --> Leads have to first find out you exist
- **LIKE & TRUST** --> Over time they come to like and trust you and your gym
- **HIRE** --> Eventually they respond to offers to take action

Lead generation starts with creating awareness about your gym.

NOTE: Do not attempt to do every single one of these lead generation strategies. The hard part of running a gym is deciding how to use a finite amount of time, energy, and money.

For help in deciding what to do next in a given week, month, or quarter, it's often helpful to get an outside eye.

Want help? Business for Unicorns offers free 10-minute brainstorm calls for gym owners.

*Go to **BusinessForUnicorns.com/Brainstorm***

OR use the QR code below to book your call today.

☐ Organized Email Database

Before we look for *new* leads, we start by organizing your existing list of contacts.

Right now, there may be people with whom you already have a relationship that may not know you have a gym. These people already **KNOW, LIKE,** and **TRUST** you. So this is the first place we start marketing our services.

Anyone you would say hi to in the grocery store should be aware you own a gym. And they should hear from you on a regular basis so they don't forget!

To organize your contacts:

- Choose an Email Service Provider like Mailchimp, ConvertKit, or ActiveCampaign.
- Review your email contact list. Upload anyone who meets the above criteria.
- Review your cell phone contacts and look for anyone else to add. If you don't have their email, text them and ask them.
- If you are using a booking and billing platform for your gym, upload these contacts too.
- Create different "segments" by tagging them based on your relationship
  - Current Clients
  - Former Clients
  - Never-Been-Clients
  - Family and Friends

Send your list of to-be-added contacts a warm-up email from your personal email. Let them know you'd like to keep them up to date with what's happening at your gym. Assure them it's ok to unsubscribe if they'd rather not hear from you.

We'll discuss what kind and frequency of emails to send in **LEAD NURTURE SYSTEMS** later in the book. But the first step is making sure you have a comprehensive email list.

PRO TIP: Use an email address with your gym's URL. This is important for professionalism AND deliverability.

Ex. *mark@markfisherfitness.com NOT hotbunz@aol.com*

☐ Referral Systems

Getting warm introductions from your clients is one of the best ways for people to find out about you.

There are two kinds of referral systems. You'll need each of them for best results.

1) Evergreen Referral Offer

Your Evergreen Referral Offer is always available. It has two components:

- Something valuable and easy for your client to give away (e.g. a free session)
- A way to thank your client for referring (e.g. a card and/or $50 credit)

We want to make it EASY for your clients to refer. Consider creating a landing page for them to input their friends' contact info. You could also create one for them to send to their friend to claim their valuable gift.

We're not looking to drive behavior with an incentive. Most clients won't take different actions because of a credit. But we ARE looking to express gratitude to clients who help grow your business.

The Evergreen Referral offer won't drive behavior in and of itself. But building referral asks into your business *will*. Identify key times to ask for a referral, including but not limited to:

- Bringing a friend to the Strategy Session
- Bringing a friend to their first workout
- Offering a free session or trial for a friend at the end of a prospect's trial
- On a member's anniversary
- Reminding your entire member base about the evergreen offer via

    - An email campaign
    - Announcements before sessions
    - Posts in a members' Facebook Group
    - Physical flyers in the space

2) Referral Campaign Offer

In addition to your Evergreen Referral Offer, consider a dedicated Referral Campaign 2-4 times per year.

You can test a number of different campaigns so you find what works best. Plus you won't burn out your clients by always doing the same thing. Some of the most popular options are:

- Bring-a-Buddy Week - Members can bring a friend to work out for free for an entire week (either with or without them).
- Free Trial/Month - Members can give away 14-30 days of your services to a friend.
- Give-to-Get Contest - Members participate in a contest and earn points for activities that grow your business. Examples include:

- Posting on social media
- Submitting contact info for friends
- Getting friends to come to a work out
- Getting friends to sign up for a trial
- Leaving a review

☐ Business Partnerships

Another way to grow your audience is by partnering with other businesses.

Here are the core tools you'll need for this system:

☐ Give & Get List - Make a menu of all the things you could *give* to a business partner and all the things you could *get* from a business partner. Examples include sending a dedicated email, doing a social media post, hanging a flyer, highlighting a "business of the month," free or discounted services for the other owner and/or their team, participating in a charity or community event for each others' business, etc.

☐ A List of Possible Partners - There are two main categories here:

- DEMOgraphic Partners - These businesses share your avatar. Usually health and fitness related, like a chiropractor, athletic wear, or a supplement store.
- GEOgraphic Partners - These businesses are located close to your gym, but may not be explicitly related to health and fitness.

Examples include a coffee shop, a brewery, or a local clothing boutique.

- ○ NOTE: Clients who also own businesses can be great partners.

☐ Business Partner Tracker - Once you have your list, make contact with at least 1-2 new businesses per month. Keep notes for your contacts and how you'll help each others' business. In addition to adding new partners each month, *keep up with your existing partners.* Touch base at least once per month. Be a friend!

When starting the relationship, give them a call or email in advance. Let them know you'd love to connect. Stop by with coffee. If appropriate, make purchases from them. Be persistent and patient!

To do Business Partnerships well, **always start with a giving hand.** Focus first on being friendly. Focus second on how you can help them. Only then start to offer ways they can help you. And remember, this is a long game. Don't expect this to drive tons of leads overnight!

PRO TIP: Although not technically a business partnership, don't forget about local organizations like teachers, the police department, the fire department, etc. These can be great groups to grow awareness in the community.

☐ Live Events

Another way to grow your audience is through live events. This can look a lot of different ways based on your gym and the event in question. But there's real value in showing up everywhere.

The most common strategy is a table at a health fair, farmer's market, 5k race, or an event for your town. The key to success is a visually compelling presence AND a way to get contact information. Having something small to give away (like branded chapstick) can be nice. But it's even better to get contact info. Consider running contests, games, or raffles for a free trial or membership that require getting email addresses.

Besides *other people's events*, you can also host your OWN events.

Community events for your gym can be a great way to meet your clients' friends. Events can also grow a shared audience with participating business partners. Depending on your market and culture, examples could include:

- Having a team at an athletic event like a mud run or 5k
- A "lunch and learn" workshop for a local business
- A party at a local brewery
- An event in your gym
- A game night
- A picnic
- A hike

There are MANY ways to run events and generate more leads for your gym. Just remember, for this to be valuable, it has to be more than mere brand awareness.

Get contact information so you can add to your email database. Now that they **KNOW** you, email them over time so they come to **LIKE & TRUST** you, and eventually respond to offers to **HIRE** you.

This is mostly a long tail game. But a handful of prospects may already be in the market for a gym. Consider making a time sensitive offer to new leads to take action and **HIRE** you.

NOTE: While not technically a Live Event, another place to build awareness is local Facebook Groups. Depending on the group and its focus, it may or may not be appropriate to directly market your business. At the least, you can build more local relationships and be friendly and helpful. In some cases, it may even be acceptable to post offers to learn more about your gym.

☐ Paid Marketing

A full accounting of paid resources is beyond the scope of this book. But all mature gyms should consider paid lead acquisition.
At the time of this writing, Meta (Facebook & Instagram) ads are still king. They're more expensive than ever. And the leads are colder than ever. But well-executed follow-up and sales will still convert enough to make it worth it.

Google Ads can also be a powerful source of lead generation. They're more expensive and won't replicate the volume of Meta ads. But they can play an important role in prospects finding you when they're searching for a solution. This is because the leads are "higher intent." Unlike Meta, these leads are searching for keywords related to your fitness solution. Related, YouTube ads can be effective in many markets.

Paid *digital* ads are a key pillar when looking for scale. But you may want to consider other paid lead generation systems:

- Direct Mail - Spam mail has evolved into a mostly digital (e-mail) animal. This means you can take advantage of relatively spartan "snail" mailboxes. Further, direct mail allows you to send postcards to a precisely chosen set of addresses near your gym. You can even target by demographic details like income. The key here is remembering this audience is cold. This means:

    - You'll need a well-designed postcard with a very strong offer to get them to take action
    - You'll need to do *at least* three mailings 30 days apart

- Sponsorships - Sponsorships are similar to business partnerships. Unlike business partnerships, they are a direct quid pro quo. You're paying cash for explicitly promoting your business. The most valuable sponsorships will let you send offers to their emails list. The least valuable sponsorships merely stick your logo on things like jerseys or websites. This latter category is not worth your time.

- Traditional Advertising - Finally, there are a number of traditional forms of paid marketing to consider.

Examples include advertising in a local newspaper, local magazine, local radio, a billboard, etc. The right ad in the right place with the right offer can still work magic. Be sure to create a specific offer, url, and/or phone number to track results. Just be warned: when you DON'T get this right, this can easily become a cash drain with no return.

☐ Ground Game "Meeting and Greeting"

This is perhaps the least sexy and most underrated strategy for getting the word out about your gym.

The above strategies are great. It makes sense to generate leads through your existing network, clients, and business partners. And being able to pay for leads is also important.

But at the end of the day, nothing replaces good ol' getting out in the community and meeting people. Your core goal is to *obliterate obscurity*. So spend time meeting strangers in your community and telling them about your gym. You could go into a local coffee shop and buy people coffee (with business cards) as they come in. You could walk around a local community event introducing yourself. You could greet people in the parking lot of a nearby strip mall or grocery store or Target. You could go buy coffees (with business cards) to give away to parents waiting to pick up their kids after school.

You'll want to use social intuition about when and how you do this. And in fact, there will be situations where you may even be asked to stop. But very few gym owners overdo this strategy. Most gym owners are unwilling to promote their services to strangers in-person. And this hamstrings their success.

To do this well:

- Create a special QR code that drives to a unique URL with a special "Neighbor" offer. This will let you track results.
- Create a well-designed business card or flyer with the special offer and a QR code to give away.
- Consider an extra incentive for anyone willing to give you contact information. This is far more valuable than just giving away cards/flyers. But it's a harder "sell."
- Create and track a weekly target for business cards given away. You can also track contacts obtained.
- Enroll your team in helping. Train them well and provide and roleplay a script. Give them time to do it and a target number per week.

LEAD NURTURE SYSTEMS

You now have a growing audience of people who **KNOW** you exist. Next, we'll develop a relationship with them so they **LIKE & TRUST** you.

We will build good will by providing valuable content via email and social media. This content will:

- Educate - Help them solve problems and answer common fitness questions
- Entertain - Give them an enjoyable experience via the content or the way it's delivered
- Encourage - Inspire them to achieve their goals and motivate them to take action

NOTE: Another way to build trust is by creating "omni-presence." If you're building awareness of your gym with the **Lead Generation Systems**, they'll see your gym everywhere. This repeated exposure will in and of itself create **LIKE & TRUST.** Psychologists call this the *"Mere Exposure Effect."*

☐ Email Marketing

You now have a well-organized email database. Next, you will regularly email valuable content that builds **LIKE & TRUST** over time.

Most gyms should target at least one email per week. If you have the bandwidth to create enough high-quality content, this can be scaled up to three times per week.

Here are two more email marketing tools to add to your arsenal.

☐ Content Ideas List - Make a list in a Google Doc of the most common problems your avatar faces and the most common questions they ask. Be sure to use *the words they actually use.* Then create content that provides solutions and answers.

☐ Email Marketing Content Calendar - Create a Google Doc to draft your emails. Get at least four weeks ahead so you have a buffer when life inevitably happens. Be consistent with your marketing. *Don't break the chain!* By planning ahead, you can also be proactive when you layer in direct sales messaging and promos. More about this in the **Marketing Calendar** section later in the book.

There's a LOT to say about email marketing. Things like design, readability, and subject lines all matter. And depending on your approach, integrating personal stories will humanize your business. But to start, the most important element is staying consistent.

PRO TIP: Every email needs to make it clear *exactly what your prospects should do next* when they're ready to take action. Sending out email content without clarifying next steps is a missed opportunity. At the same time, you don't want to always hammer sales messaging.

The best way to split the difference is using something called the "Super Signature" (h/t to marketing legend Dean Jackson). The PS is the most read part of your email. Always use the PS as a CTA for the next step for interested prospects.

Here's an example. (Note the word "TODAY" would be hyperlinked to a booking calendar.)

> *PS: Would you like to work with us to achieve your fitness goals?*
>
> *Whenever you're ready, your very first step is a no-pressure, 10-minute Discovery Call. We'll ask you a few questions and tell you more about our absolutely no-risk trial.*
>
> *Book your call **TODAY**.*

☐ Instagram Content System

At the time of this writing, Instagram is the most valuable organic social media platform. Instagram allows you to nurture your followers so they **LIKE & TRUST** you. But by tagging and collaborating with your clients and team, you can also be discovered by new people. This makes Instagram unique. It can both drive awareness so people **KNOW** you exist AND build **LIKE & TRUST** over time.

- ☐ Profile with a Clear CTA - Think of your Instagram profile as a secondary website. Just like your website, it should be immediately clear 1) Who you help 2) How you help them and 3) Exactly what to do next.

  Your CTA can drive to the link in your profile for the action you want prospects to take. In most cases, this will be a Low Barrier Offer.

- ☐ Instagram Marketing Content Calendar - Just like email marketing, plan your Instagram content in advance. You can use the same Content Ideas list you use for emails. And just like emails, you'll want to get out at least several weeks ahead.

  Consider batching your content creation. Shoot for at least 3 Feed Posts per week and 1-3 Stories per day. Experiment with different kinds of content. See what your audience responds to best and what you most enjoy creating. And remember, just like with email, all content should have a CTA.

WARNING: Instagram can become an unprofitable time suck for many gym owners. Not only might you get distracted by consuming content, you can also end up spending lots of time posting with no results.

While you do need to be on Instagram, the only non-negotiable is that the gym is active enough that it looks open. Use compelling photos of your gym in action, with real pics of your clients. Share value-building content that Educates, Entertains, and Encourages.

But don't feel pressured to be an "Influencer." It's ok to put Instagram on a simmer if you don't enjoy it and you don't get the best returns on your time. Just be sure the effort you DO put in drives gym growth.

For more about how to use Instagram to build relationships and make offers, check out **Sell By Chat** later in the book.

☐ **Client Case Study Systems**

Client testimonials and Google Reviews are important tools to build **LIKE & TRUST**. You can use Instagram and emails to deliver proof of positive clients experiences. You can display them on your website. You can build ad campaigns that drive colder audiences to watch testimonial videos. And you can even share them in your prospect follow-up.

The best client stories have three parts:

1. The challenges and frustrations of life BEFORE working with your gym
2. The moment when they realized your gym was helping create change, often coupled with a specific set of behaviors

3. The specific results and positive feelings of life AFTER working with your gym

You'll need two different kinds of Client Case Study Systems:

☐ Testimonial Capture System - This is best captured by video. You can then create:

- A well-edited 60-90 second video
- A templated pull quote with a picture of a client looking happy and healthy

☐ Google Reviews System - Getting Google Reviews will provide social proof when prospects research you. They will also improve your ranking in search results. You'll need a system to get your clients to leave Google Reviews by asking at key points in their customer journey.

Examples of places to ask for a Google Review include:

- At the end of their first 4 weeks
- Any time a client talks positively about their experience
- Once every 6 months via a mass email campaign to all clients
- In flyers with QR codes posted at your gym
- When otherwise happy clients need to terminate their membership

☐ Other Lead Nurture Platforms

Over time, other platforms may become important to brick and mortar gym owners. Gyms with sufficient capacity can consider experimenting with a YouTube channel, a podcast, or a TikTok presence.

Just be sure to prioritize the other strategies first. At current these platforms are not the best place for brick and mortar businesses to grow their audience. In some limited cases, they could be useful for lead nurture. But only IF the owner has the capacity, talent, and interest to create great content here.

Specifically, podcasts can be a great *retention* tool by interviewing clients. In turn, your clients may share their interview, which could lead to more referrals. Related, interviewing other local small business owners could deepen your relationship with possible business partners. They may also share their interview with their business's audience.

Finally, some gyms may want to experiment with creating a private Facebook Group geared towards prospects.

Like emails and Instagram, this could be one more channel to build **LIKE & TRUST** with leads. You can post valuable resources and ask questions to spark engagement. And you can make offers to a captive audience. However, at the time of this writing, Facebook Groups no longer have quite the traction they did a few years ago. Furthermore, it will require effort (and possibly paid ads) to grow a Facebook Group of local leads. Then it will be one more digital platform that requires ongoing time and attention. So be sure you have the bandwidth before you decide to test this strategy. There may be lower hanging fruit.

LEAD CONVERSION SYSTEMS

Our leads now **KNOW** who we are and are coming to **LIKE & TRUST** us. Next we'll invite them to take the next step to work with us.

We've already built your offer. We're showcasing it on your website and Instagram profile. We've also started to share it via email marketing, Instagram posts, paid ads, or other channels.

Now we need a system to follow-up with those who've expressed interest. Most people won't follow through without support.

Finally, we'll need a structured conversation to clarify their goals and explain your gym's value. Only then will we invite them to commit to a membership.

☐ **Sell By Chat Script**

Too often, Instagram is a place for erratically posting content. We need a reliable way to turn your audience into actual leads and clients.

By starting conversations in DMs, you can build a relationship more quickly. In some cases, you can move people right into an offer. Just keep in mind, most people won't be ready to move that fast. Yes, you do want to identify leads ready to take action. But it's important to go into DM convos with the intention to build a relationship and be helpful.

Although you can do specific Feed Posts and Stories to invite engagement, a simple trigger is to start a conversation with anyone who is following you.

A good "Sell by Chat" script will have four sections:

1. Conversation Openers - This is an easy-to-answer question to start the conversation. The goal here is simply to get a response. Classic examples include:

    - *"Thanks for the follow! How did you hear about me?"*
    - *"Thanks for the follow! Are you just here for the content or are you interested in [X fitness goal]?"*
    - *"Thanks for commenting on my post! Do you live in [neighborhood]?"*

2. Connection Builders - Continue the conversation by asking simple "this or that" questions. Your new friend will be able to answer without having to think too hard. At this point we're breaking the ice and establishing rapport. Examples include:

    - *"Do you know anyone at our gym?"*
    - *"Do you have a specific goal you're working towards or just general health?"*
    - *"Do you have a current fitness routine that you like?"*

3. Qualifying Questions - At a certain point, we need to find out if this individual is a viable lead. As a gym owner, you don't have the luxury of having lots of conversations that don't lead anywhere. After a few "this or that" questions, you can dig in a bit deeper to see if they're a fit for your services. Examples include:

   - *"Thinking about your goal of [X]... what would you say you need most to get there?"*
   - *Thinking about your goal of [X]... what would you say is the biggest barrier: time, motivation, or knowledge?"*

4. Offer Makers - Finally, it's time to make an offer for next steps. The best offer here is a 10-minute brainstorm. If you know they're a qualified candidate for your services, this is well worth your time. You can then follow the Discovery Call script (see below) to move them into your front end offer. If you have a very low barrier offer (like a free class), you may be able to offer it here as well.

   - *"Would you like some help with that?"*
   - *"Here's what I'm thinking…"*
   - *"We can set up a 10-minute brainstorm on [specific problem] and map out a plan to [achieve goal]."*
   - *"You up for that?"*

If possible, do the call then and there. If not, offer them two times in the next 24 hours to schedule.

Remember, Sell By Chat won't always lead to a sale right away. Be patient. Build some rapport, be friendly, and be helpful. Follow up on conversations that go cold. Keep the relationship alive!

AND on the other hand… there comes a time to make an ask. We put this tool in **Lead Conversion Systems** because you DO want to make offers via DM. Don't get friend zoned. If you're having lots of long convos that aren't going anywhere? Review your script. Look for places to move from Connection Building to Qualifying Question and Offer Makers.

☐ Follow-Up Systems

Follow-Up Systems are the single most neglected gym sales and marketing tool.

There's nothing more tragic than doing tons of work to generate leads… *only to ignore those leads.*

There are two reasons that follow-ups fall off.

1) Some gym owners don't want to be pushy.

This makes sense. No one wants to be a used car salesman. But this is someone who has explicitly expressed interest. Furthermore, an oft-quoted internet stat says 80% of all purchases happen on the 5th to 12th touch. And whether this is from actual data, any seasoned gym owner will tell you the spirit is correct.

Finally, it's not only good business, but *good coaching* to follow up with them until they take action. Keep reaching out until they tell you they're no longer interested.

2) Some gym owners don't have systems in place to organize their lead follow-up.

In some cases the gym owner *wants* to do more follow-up. But they're just too busy and disorganized to give follow-up the attention it deserves.

A good lead management software will be part of the solution. A small gym with limited lead flow can get by on spreadsheets for a while. But at some point you'll need software with automations and task assignments. This will streamline your daily lead follow-up.

You can set up your software to launch automations after your leads express interest.

In most cases, the very first step will be:

1. An opt-in form on a landing page or paid ad for a front end barrier offer
2. An opt-in form when booking a phone call to learn more

This is why it's best to "gate" the first step by asking for First Name, Phone Number, and Email *first*. If they "abandon cart" and don't finish booking their call or purchasing the LBO, you can follow up with them.

NOTE: One of the most important elements in successful follow up is *speed*. The use of automations is very important here. No matter when they take action, you can set up automated email and text message follow-up. This will keep them moving along to your next step (usually setting up a call). Having said that, you'll get even better results if you can call them within 5 minutes of opting in.

Once you have software in place, you'll need to decide your exact follow-up system.

- **Frequency** - How often will you follow-up with your leads? As a general rule, you'll want *at least* 15-20 total touches over the first 14 days after a lead expresses interest. This can be front-loaded with 2-4 touches per day (via different channels) in the first 48 hours.

- **Channels** - Use different channels for your outreach. Different people will respond to different communications. Text messages, phone calls, and emails should all be a part of your follow-up. Plus by varying your channels, you'll be less annoying.

- **Scripts** - Finally, you'll need to have a script so you know what to say. When in doubt, keep it simple. Be a human. Acknowledge that you don't want to be annoying, but you know life gets busy. Consider sharing some testimonials in your outreach.

Proper lead follow-up can feel overwhelming. But the good news is this: if you simply follow-up consistently with all leads, you'll be in the top 1% of gyms.

Resist the temptation to over-analyze here. There's no magic sequence of follow-up frequency, channels, or scripts. Just make sure you hit *at least* 15-20 touches over the first 14 days.

After this 14-day window, the lead will continue to get your email marketing. This will build more **LIKE & TRUST** and allow you to make more offers. You can also do dedicated offers specifically to leads who took action but never made contact. (See more on this topic in the **Marketing Calendar** section.)

PRO TIP: You'll also need a system to follow-up with leads *after they've made an appointment.* Part of your follow-up will be reminders about your upcoming sales appointment. This can be automated. Send these out the day before and/or day of. Consider doing a personalized video showing off your space and humanizing yourself. You'll also need a dedicated follow-up system for when someone no-shows.

A final note about appointment availability…

One of the most important factors in successful conversion to booking sales appointments is *availability.* Gym owners are often very busy because we wear a lot of hats. But if you can only do sales appointments on Fridays at 2pm, don't expect your business to grow.

In particular for Discovery Call calendars, you want a short, wide open window. This means don't let people book more than 3-5 days out, and have as much availability as you can realistically manage at different times of day.

☐ **Sales Scripts**

To be successful at sales, you ***need a script.*** You've done a lot of work to generate and nurture leads. The final step is to get **HIRED.** And it's too important to wing it.

I'm not suggesting you read a script like a robot. There will always be a place for "humanizing the system." But the only way to achieve consistent success is by repeatedly executing a well-choreographed sales conversation. This is all the more important if you want anyone else on your team to handle sales appointments.

Some people bristle at using a script. But let's be honest. You already tend to say the same things over and over. This system is about creating clarity on the very best phrases and questions to create the best results.

Most gyms will need two different scripts.

- [ ] Discovery Phone Call Script - This 10-minute introductory call is the first step a lead takes when they're exploring **HIRING** you. Depending on your model, you will "sell" them and set them up with a free or paid front end offer. In some cases, this call will be used to book a follow-up strategy session before anything is sold. The Discovery Call can be scheduled in advance with a booking link. Or it can happen spontaneously when you're calling leads and they pick up the phone.

- [ ] Strategy Session Script - This is a 30-45 minute conversation where you sell memberships. In some cases, you may sell a mid or high ticket front end offer as your first step. In this longer conversation you'll go deeper into your prospects' underlying WHY behind their goals. In general, the Strategy Session will have four parts:

1. Break the Ice - Build rapport. Find out how they heard about you. Lay out exactly what's going to happen and how long it will take.

2. Peel the Onion - Clarify their most important goals. Dig into why it's important to them and how their life will change. Identify obstacles that have gotten in the way of success in the past.

3. Build Value - Explain how your services create the outcomes they want (in the words they used). Explain how your services overcome previous obstacles (in the words they used). This can take the form of a verbal explanation, a tour of the gym, an assessment, a brief workout, or some combination.

   - PRO TIP: Only talk about *what they care about*. Do not talk about all the benefits of your gym. Do not talk yourself out of the sale. Only talk about *what they care about.*

4. Make the Ask - Make a strong offer for the best membership for their goals. Take away all risk with a guarantee. Offer a time-sensitive attractive incentive for them to take action on the spot or by end of day.

PRO TIP: A constraint for your gym's growth is your sales availability. If you want to grow your gym but can only take sales calls at 10:30am on a Friday, you will fail.

For the Discovery Call, offer as much availability as you can, but no further than 72 hours out.

When booking a Strategy Session, book them within 24 hours whenever possible. The only exception is if you want them to sample your services *before* you make a membership offer. In that case, you will still get the Strategy Session scheduled on the Discovery Call. But you may choose to schedule it after they've already started training with you.

****

Want access to BFU's proven done-for-you sales scripts?

*You can pick up ours at **BusinessForUnicorns.com/Sales***

OR by using the QR code below

MARKETING PLANNING SYSTEMS

We now know how to:

- Grow your list of leads who **KNOW** your gym
- Build a relationship so they **LIKE & TRUST** you over time
- Invite prospects to **HIRE** you and become a client

But we have one final set of systems that brings together all the other systems.

"A To Do list that doesn't exist in a time is a recipe for being miserable/sad/crazy." - Me

Too many gym owners get this far and get overwhelmed. These final two systems allow you to plan out what you will do each day, week, month, and quarter. They will organize the above tools into a *schedule* so you know what to do and when to grow your gym.

☐ **Marketing Calendar**

Many gym owners know they should have a marketing calendar. But they get too overwhelmed to actually take action.

In practice, a good marketing calendar for your gym is *simple*. It should be pretty high level. Marketing calendars have two core components.

1) A detailed calendar for the next three months.

2) A crude calendar for what happens over the rest of the calendar year.

Since you'll want some flexibility, you don't need to worry about a detailed plan for an entire year ahead. That said, you DO want to know exactly what's happening in the next three months. In fact, if this all feels like a lot? You can even get away with simply planning out three months at a time and not worry about the rest of the year.

Here's the simplest way to think about this:

For each of the next three months, you can do one offer or message for one or more of the main three segments of your audience (Current Clients, Former Clients, Never-Been Clients). You can decide what to offer or message based on the time of year, a holiday, or even internal milestones like gym anniversaries or your birthday.

NOTE: I'm using the word "message" as well as "offers." Because in some situations, it may not be a literal offer. For example, for your Current Clients, you may choose to ask for referrals or a Google Review. This isn't an offer per se. But you'll still want to be strategic in how and when you make this ask. Other examples of non-offer messages include promoting an event for a business partnership, a charity bootcamp, or anything else you want to highlight to your community.

The calendar itself can be a simple Google Doc. If you want to get fancy, you can use a spreadsheet. You could also consider using a big whiteboard in an office if your gym has one.

There's a balance to be struck when planning your marketing calendar. If you do too much messaging and too often, your audience will tune out. On the other hand, if you don't make offers frequently enough, you won't grow as fast as you could.

Besides the calendar itself, you'll also want a list of possible offers and messages to test. This way you're not starting from scratch each time you plan your next three months.

Most offers/messages are best promoted in a 10-14 day window. If you go too long, it becomes noise. If you go too short, you won't have time to properly promote it.

Finally, when you DO promote something, market FULL-OUT across all channels.

If you're going to market… MARKET!

You don't need (or want) to use all these channels every time. Different offers/messages for different markets will have different strategies. But to jog your brain, here's a list of options to consider:

- Bulk Email Marketing
- Individual Emails
- Bulk Text Messages
- Individual Text Messages
- Phone Calls
- Organic Social Media Posts & Stories
- Updated Instagram Profile
- Class or Sessions Announcements
- Flyers in the Gym with CTAs and QR Codes
- Posts in a Private Facebook Group
- Updated Website Homepage Messaging

- Promotion from Business Partners to their Audience
- Physical Mailing

****

Want access to BFU's list of the very best offers for your gym to consider?

*You can pick up ours at **BusinessForUnicorns.com/Offers***

OR by using the QR code below

☐ **Weekly Marketing Schedule**

Very few gym owners turn their marketing and sales activities into a *weekly calendar*. And if you miss THIS, you won't have a plan to turn all these great ideas into action.

To create your personal weekly marketing schedule, identify how many hours per week you can realistically devote. Most gym owners will need *at least* 3-5 hours per week. For more mature gyms, the gym owner may spend as much as 10-20 hours or more of their week focused on marketing and sales.

There are four main "buckets" of marketing and sales work on a daily and weekly basis:

- Building and Refining the Systems - In the beginning, much of your time will be spent "building the machine." But many of these will be one-off tasks. For instance, once you've updated your website and crafted a good LBO, you'll only need to update them once in a while.

- Lead Generation Activities - Some time each week will be spent *generating* leads so more people **KNOW** you exist. Examples include cultivating business partnerships, making referral asks, and overseeing paid digital marketing.

- Lead Nurture Activities - You will also need to build **LIKE & TRUST** over time with content marketing. Each week you will spend some time writing, sending, and posting or scheduling content. In most cases, this is best done in "batches" and not every day.

- Lead Conversion Activities - Of all the activities, this is both the most important AND the hardest to fit into prescribed times. Responsiveness and availability matter when following up with leads and doing sales appointments. You'll need to move the ball forward every workday. But the amount of time it takes will flex up and down based on how many prospects are in play.

To turn these items into a weekly schedule:

1. Decide how many hours per week you can devote
2. Schedule the hours in your calendar like you would training a session
3. *Keep your appointment!!!*

I know, I know. This is a bit anticlimactic. It seems too simple!

But in practice, this is where the vast majority of gym owners drop the ball. They get overwhelmed by putting out fires. OR they procrastinate because they don't like marketing and sales.

To that last point… this makes sense! It's hard to like something you know you're not good at (yet).

Commit to doing the work here. Just like you'd counsel your clients, focus on the process at first. Get in your "bad reps" while you build skill. Over time your results will improve, your confidence will increase, and you may even come to enjoy the activities that grow your business!

THANK YOU FOR READING!

There you have it, my Gym Owner friend.

The world's simplest and most comprehensive approach to marketing your gym.

No more frustrating lead trickle. No more flailing around doing random "marketing stuff." No more weeks with no sales appointments!

You CAN create a steady stream of interested and qualified prospects. You can have the piece of mind that comes from knowing you're getting traction. And when you get this right, you'll have a growing base of happy clients and revenues that increase month over month.

I've written this little book to point you in the right direction. And you may be ready to go take action. Which is great!

But I know some percentage of readers will want more support in deciding what order to tackle this in.

And frankly, no matter how ready you are to take action…

You'll save lots of time — and make lots more money — if you have a *customized order of operations* for your gym and your situation.

I'd love to invite you to hop on a *free 10-minute brainstorming session* with me or someone on my team.

In this fast-paced call, we'll get clear on:

- The results you want to achieve in the next 90 days and beyond
- The #1 roadblock restricting your gym's growth and holding you back
- A clear 3-Step Plan to get you results in your gym ASAP

Go to ***BusinessForUnicorns.com/Brainstorm*** or use the QR code below to book your call today.

I hope you've found this book has created some clarity for you. And looking forward to staying in touch!

Much love,
Mark and the BFU Team

LET'S STAY IN TOUCH!

I think we've got a good thing going here, yeah? ;-)

If you agree, I'd love to stay in touch.

You can find a ton of free resources on our website. And if you like this book, I bet you'll love our YouTube channel and podcast.

If you want to know more about me or Business for Unicorns, here are some places to check us out:

- BusinessForUnicorns.com
- MarkFisherYouTube.com
- BFUPodcast.com
- BusinessForUnicorns.com/Book

The last URL will take you to another book I wrote. It's a bunch of lessons and stories from my 10-plus years running MFF.

And if you want a FREE digital copy?

Message us on Instagram at **@businessforunicorns** and we'll get you one!

Want even *more* BFU in your life?

Follow us on Instagram for
more strategies to build a gym and life you love.

@businessforunicorns